Keto Meal Prep Cookbook

Keto Meal Prep Recipes The Complete Proven Guide To Rapid Weight Loss and Save Time With 14-Days Keto Meal Plan

By [Kathy Robinson]

Table of Contents

Introduction 1

The Essential Knowledge Keto Diet Meal Prep? 2

What is Ketogenic diet? 2

9 Wonderful Benefits of Keto Diet you'll find in the next few weeks 4

7 Big advantages of the Meal prep you will want in your life 6

Does A Low-Carb keto diet really work? 7

There are 7 signs and Symptoms that You're in ketosis 9

The 5 Most Important Common Mistakes in Keto Diet Meal Prep 10

6 Proven Tips That will Help You Make The Best Keto Meal Prep Journey 11

The Top 20 Foods Need to Avoid 12

Over 30 Delicious Foods You can eat 14

Yummy Breakfast Recipes to Start Your Morning Right 17

Sausage and Egg Muffin 17

Breakfast Loaf with Berry and Peanut Butter 19

Keto Cereal 21

Ham and Cheese Waffles 22

Baked Eggs with Avocado 24

Cheese, Egg and Bacon Cups 25

Yoghurt Parfait 26

Salad with chicken breast and spinach 27

Bacon lemon thyme breakfast muffins 28

Cheese omelet with bacon 29

Easy to Make Lunch Meals 30

Buffalo Chicken Lettuce Wraps 30

Beef Burritos 34

Open-Faced Prosciutto and Brie Sandwich with Avocado Bun 36

Keto Cubano 37

Keto Monkey Bread 38

Cauliflower Grits With Roasted Mushrooms And Walnuts 39

Crispy Pork Salad 42

Dinner Is Never Boring with These Water-Mouthing Meals **45**

Cauliflower Taboule Salad 45

Thai Chicken with cauliflower rice 47

Grilled chicken skewers with garlic sauce 49

Pasta with chicken and basil 51

Salmon Fishcakes 52

Baby back Ribs 53

Garlic Cream Pork Chops 56

Spaghetti Carbonara 57

Shrimp in Tuscan Cream Sauce 58

Delightful Snacks Meals **59**

Herb Dressed Chicken Parmesan Fingers 59

Bacon Moza Sticks 61

Buffalo Chicken Dip 62

Choco Berry Protein Bars 63

Amazing Chipotle Kale Chips 64

Simple Fine Granola 65

Raspberry and Cheesy Pops 66

Buffalo Drumsticks 67

Satisfying Tuna Croquettes 68

Deep Walnut Bites 69

Amazing Dessert Meals **70**

Pumpkin and Cardamom Donuts 70

Blueberry Morning Scones 72

Poppy Seed Juicy Cupcake 75

Raspberry Popsicles 76

Secret Yogurt Parfait 77

Choco Peanut Fat Bombs 78

Creamy Vanilla Pudding 79

Pretty Pizza Fat Bombs 80

14-Days Keto Meal Plan for Rapid Fat Loss With 2-Weeks Healthy Shopping List 81

Conclusion 87

Introduction

Congratulations on purchasing this book and thank you for doing so.

The following chapters will discuss what a ketogenic diet is and how it can benefit you and your lifestyle.

The Keto Diet is one that builds on a number of previous ideas around the value of a low carb high fat food intake, and this focus is a well-established idea. There is a lot of evidence that the Keto diet can provide quick results in terms of **weight loss**, **energy improvements**, and **healthy living** in general. These meals really focus on healthy, and tasty, eating.

By reading the prepping section of the book, finding your own prepping day or days, planning meals carefully and shopping sensibly, you really will s**ave time and money while enjoying fresh tasting**, vibrant meals that will make cooking a joy and eating a thrill.

Prepping can change your life. Seriously. Having food ready to heat and eat means that you avoid that dilemma of whether to cook or get a take out. Everything is there, in the fridge, ready to go. The quickest option is to eat in, with your own freshly cooked food. This will eliminate a lot of temptations that lead you away from your dietary goals.

Included in these chapters are ketogenic recipes as well as a 14-day menu on foods that can be portioned and prepped, as well as a section on common ketogenic and food prep misconceptions and concerns.

There are several books related to this subject on the market, thanks again for choosing this one! Every effort was made to ensure it is full of as much useful information as possible, please enjoy!

The Essential Knowledge Keto Diet Meal Prep?

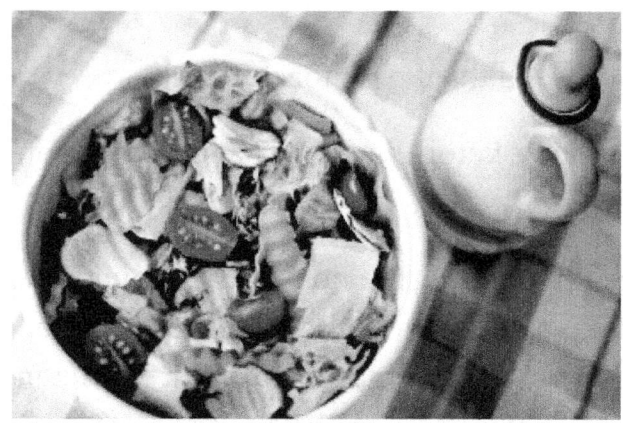 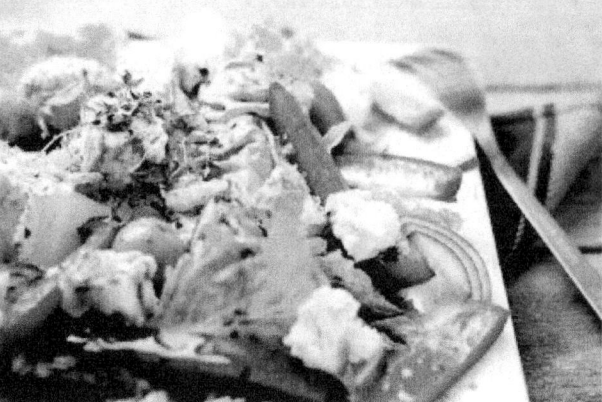

The word Ketogenic is getting a lot of hype these days and comes to the lime light more often than before. Since the whole diet plan of our book is based on a Ketogenic lifestyle, we will dive deeper to expand your understanding of the Ketogenic Diet.

What is Ketogenic diet?

A ketogenic diet is a form of low carb diet. It is characterized by an extremely low carbohydrate and very high-fat diet. Due to the lack of carbohydrates, the metabolism changes and gets into the so-called "ketosis".

Normally, the body gains energy from the dietary carbohydrates - so it depends on carbohydrate intake. If these carbohydrates are lacking as an energy source, the body needs to help elsewhere.

In the liver, fats are then converted into so-called ketone bodies, which are used instead of carbohydrates to generate energy and, for example, maintain the brain's capacity. This state of energy production is called "ketosis" and is the principle on which the ketogenic diet is based.

During a ketogenic diet, energy needs should be met as follows:

• Carbohydrates: 5 percent

- Proteins: 35 percent

- Fat: 60 percent

"Very low carbs, high in fat, limited in protein" - that's the recipe of the ketogenic diet. A ketogenic diet is nothing more than a strict low carb, more precisely low carb high fat diet, in which the protein content is kept in moderation for a reason.

A ketogenic diet (often simply called "keto") is a diet with a very low level of carbohydrates that puts the body in the state of highest fat burning. The entire organism derives its energy in the ketogenic diet almost exclusively from the metabolism of fat. The level of insulin in the blood is constantly low in the ketogenic diet. This makes it easy for the body to access body fat reserves in addition to dietary fat.

The ketogenic diet has many powerful health benefits. Fortunately, more and more of them are currently coming to light and will be published. A ketogenic diet is a safe way to lose weight and reduce body fat. And it can increase mental and physical performance and endurance, as the energy supply of fat metabolism is safer and more even than carbohydrate metabolism. Because this fluctuates quickly and often the blood sugar level. Fat, on the other hand, is almost always available and burns more slowly.

Energy production in the ketogenic diet is similar to conventional primary energy production from carbohydrates like a coal-fired oven compared to a campfire.

However, a ketogenic diet also has some potential side effects due to the large change in metabolism, especially at the beginning. However, these can be managed to a large extent so that just about anyone can benefit from a ketogenic diet throughout their lifetime.

For whom is ketogenic nutrition interesting?

For all…

- Men and women who want to permanently lose weight or stay slim

- People who have certain health issues, like diabetes

- People who want to prevent certain health issues and improve energy

- People who want to age slower

- Fitness fans and bodybuilders

9 Wonderful Benefits of Keto Diet you'll find in the next few weeks

A list of Health Benefits secured from a Keto Diet will be never ending. Nevertheless, for your convenience, a few of the more important health benefits that you can gain from a Keto Diet will be explained.

⊕ Big Drop in Weight Loss, Because It takes more work to turn fat into energy than it takes to turn carbs into energy.

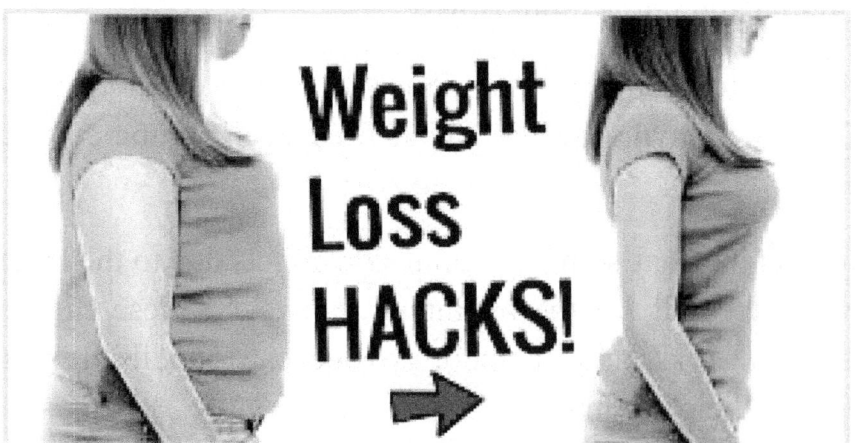

✷ A good Keto diet will help you lower the levels of bad cholesterol to prevent arterial blocks from occurring

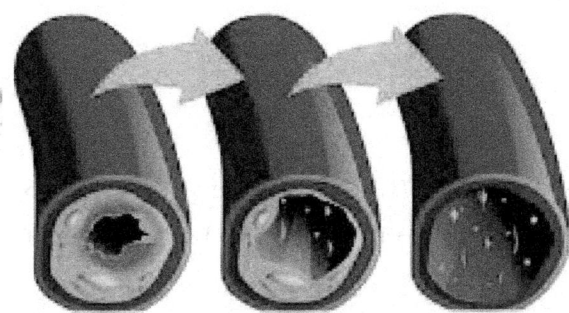

✷ Energy used by burning body fat will always keep you energetic since body fat is present in abundance in our bodies

✷ The levels of LDL will decrease which will make the body less prone to suffer from Type-2 Diabetes

✷ Decrease Your appetite, You won't always feel hungry since the diet is high in protein

✷ Ketosis helps improve skin conditions and prevents acne or skin inflammations from taking place.

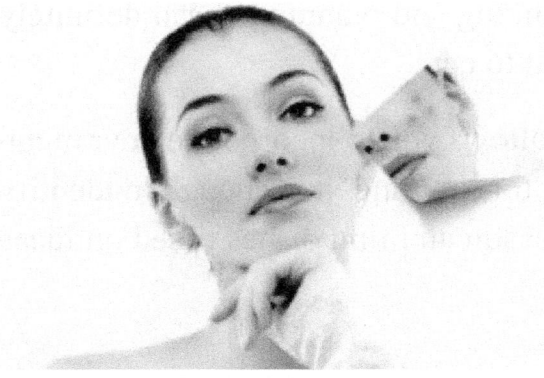

✷ Less risk for gallstones, improves digestion

🌐 Improves Mental health

🌐 Improves health in women with polycystic ovarian syndrome(PCOS)

and much more benefits are waiting for you!

7 Big advantages of the Meal prep you will want in your life

🌐 It will allow you to manage your food intake and, therefore, making it easy for you to prepare different meals in advance, knowing what to take to satisfy your caloric needs.

🌐 Meal prep will also allow you to avoid unplanned commitments and lack of time to cook as everything is ready in advance.

🌐 In addition to gaining confidence, meal prepping saves time. And yes, it allows you to go shopping less often and more efficiently since you can accurately establish the list and the exact amounts of food you will need for the entire week. It will also help you avoid wasting time, no wandering among the aisles wondering what to buy. "And if I made a quiche? Ah but no, I have no eggs..." Meal prepping will save you this dilemma.

🌐 The interest of a diet schedule of meals is diversified eating. Indeed, under the influence of pressure and hunger, we often tend to lack inspiration and opt for the same, easy, unhealthy meals. Thinking and planning ahead definitely allows you to make better choices of what to eat

🌐 Planning your meals in advance also allows you to incorporate your menu with seasonal fruits and vegetables. With this in mind, it is enough to identify the fruits and vegetables of the current season and find dishes based on ideas from them.

⊕ Managing your weekly menu with a meal prep reduces shopping on a daily basis, therefore, saving your wallet. When you shop, you only buy what you need. No more unhealthy, or unnecessary purchases.

⊕ This technique also allows you to evaluate and track your goals.

Does A Low-Carb keto diet really work?

The best way to tackle this question is to elaborate the outcome of a recent test that tackled the effectiveness of various diets when it came to shedding weight.

Technically, following a proper diet does indeed prevent gaining more weight and essentially helps our body to stay healthier.

To investigate that, in recent times a team of perhaps eight research scientists had a notion to bring into contrast the effectiveness of a Ketogenic Diet with three other different forms of diet over a period of 12 months in a completely randomized control trial. The participants of this experiment included an extensive collection of 311 individuals ranging from obese people to post-menopausal women.

Group-1 comprised of 76 people instructed to consume an Ornish Diet that had just about 10% lowered down calorie in comparison to the fatty foods.

Group 2 had 79 participants who were put on a LEARN Diet which comprised of the same 10% less calories, but this time it came from the saturated fats, while 55-60% of the calorie came from the carbohydrates. The psychological and physiological activities of this group were also monitored.

Group 3 comprising of 79 people had something called the "Zone Diet" which consisted of roughly 30%, 40% and 30% distribution of calories coming from protein, carbohydrate and fats respectively.

Finally, the last group of 77 participants was treated to a low-carb "Ketogenic" diet.

For all these diets, each subject consumed only 20 grams of carbs per day for a period of 2-3 months. After which they were directed to eat 50g per day for the coming 9-10 months.

After 12 months, the result is that all diets had shown a significant amount of reduction in BMI and overall weight alongside the percentage of body fat. However, the one that showed the maximum decline was the Ketogenic diet style.

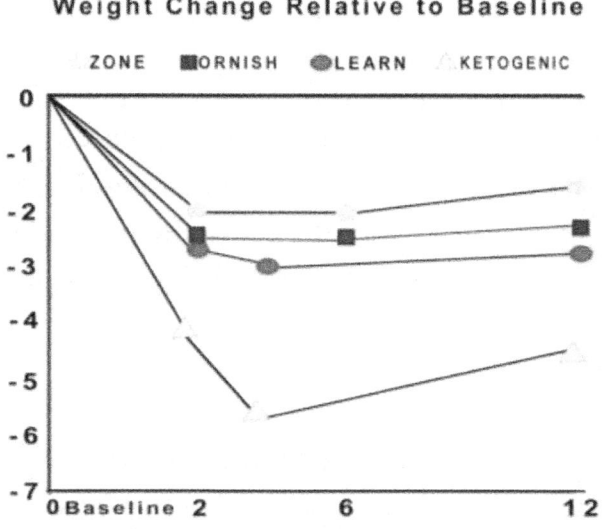

The above graph sums up the whole scenario nicely. As you can see, the decrease in BMI of the Ketogenic group is the largest. It declines a lot more than the other three diets group (LEARN group, Ornish group and Zone group).

And that's not all! Just look at the trimmed down body fat, the effects were more astonishing! The recorded decrease from the Ketogenic diet was at an astounding 7.9% while the others had a reduction of 2.5%, 2.3% and 2% in the Ornish, Zone and LEARN group respectively.

This conclusion even further supports the theory of the effectiveness of a low carb diet. In the meantime, this will help you largely to appreciate just how effective a modern Ketogenic Diet is in toning down that excess fat.

There are 7 signs and Symptoms that You're in ketosis

Apart from being able to actually test the level of Ketones by taking samples of urine, breath or blood,certain indications will help you recognize that your body is in fact in a state of ketosis. These include:

- Your mouth will feel dry and you have an increased thirst
- The number of bathroom visits will increase as you might need to urinate more often.
- Your breath will have a slight "Fruity" smell to it.
- You will get the aforementioned sensation of low levels of hunger and increased energy.
- Increased ketones, If you are in ketosis your body is producing more ketones
- Loss of appetite, but don't get hungry
- Increased focus and energy

Great, then! So, how is a person supposed to reach an optimal level of Ketosis?

It's not really as difficult as you might expect. Given that you follow a few simple rules, you will be able to thrust your body into a state of maximum Ketosis in no time!

- The first step is clearly to reduce your daily carbohydrate intake. It's better to keep it below 20 grams if possible.

- Keep the level of protein intake at moderate levels; around 70 grams if possible.

- Remember that for Ketosis to work properly, you need to maintain an ample fat intake. Make sure to eat enough fat to satisfy your body. Don't starve yourself!

- Don't have occasional snacks. Even if you are hungry; no unnecessary snacks as they might negatively affect the level of weight loss and ketosis.

The 5 Most Important Common Mistakes in Keto Diet Meal Prep

With everything said and done, it should be mentioned that there are some common mistakes that are made by new Keto enthusiasts.

- Since no proper definition of how much carb is actually "Low-Carb" exists, some people often tend to shoot their carb intake to a very high level while still considering that they are under "Low-Carb". The level of daily carb should be around 20-50 for optimal experience, but a maximum of 100-150g.

- It is understood that as macronutrient, protein is very important as a body building food. It improves the level of satiety and encourages fat burning. Yet, be aware of having too much protein as the excess might turn into glucose, which will once more be burned up for energy instead of fat.

- A very big mistake made by newcomers is they naturally think that lowering the level of fat alongside the carbs might increase the fat loss. That is absolutely wrong! Keep in mind that you need the fat in your body if you want to encourage the burning of fat!

- A key aspect when it comes to enhancing your ketogenic diet is to reduce the level of insulin. While on a ketogenic diet, your insulin levels will go down significantly, which helps greatly to relieve the level of bloat. Still, with that very process, electrolytes form our body are also flushed away. Therefore, it is essential that you balance the decrease in electrolytes by having a good amount of sodium (salt) intake to make sure that your kidneys are safe and you don't have problems such as fatigue, constipation or light headache.

The only thing left now is to know what you need and going to do, to prepare yourself for the journey ahead.

6 Proven Tips That will Help You Make The Best Keto Meal Prep Journey

- The first and foremost step is to get a carb counter guide in order to make sure that your carb intake is at desired levels.

- Open your cupboards and refrigerator and remove anything that might have a high level of carbohydrate in them, including items of whole grain.

- Restock your pantry using only low carb foods that will help you in your Keto Journey. Refer to the shopping list in the meal plan section if need be.

- Slowly and steadily give up your old habits and accept new ones that will compliment your Keto Diet

- Remember to keep plenty of drinking water nearby and always stay hydrated.

- Create and follow a strict meal plan

The Top 20 Foods Need to Avoid

Part of living a sustainable Ketogenic lifestyle involves knowing which foods to avoid. There are a lot of foods out there that some people claim to be suited for ketosis but aren't really helpful. Fortunately, ketones can be measured, which means that once you eat something, you can determine whether it has put you in ketosis or not. Luckily for you, this chapter contains a comprehensive list of foods that you need to avoid in order to achieve ketosis. This way, you don't have to keep checking your breath or urine after every meal!

Grains

All kinds of grains – including whole grains – must be avoided since they contain a high level of carbs that will prevent ketosis. Examples of such foods include:

- Wheat
- Quinoa
- Buckwheat
- Rice
- Barley
- Sorghum
- Oats
- Corn
- Amaranth
- Rye
- Millet
- Bread, pasta, cookies, pizza crusts, or crackers made from the above

Beans and Legumes

Most beans and legumes contain high starch content, so avoid the following:

- Kidney beans
- Black bean
- Pinto beans
- Lentils
- Lima beans
- Fava beans
- Chickpeas
- White beans

Fruits

- Mangos
- Papaya
- Pineapples
- Oranges
- Tangerines
- Grapes
- Fruit juices, concentrates, syrups, and smoothies

Starchy Vegetables

- Parsnips
- Potatoes
- Yams
- Yucca
- Sweet potatoes
- Carrots
- Artichoke

Alcohol

Sugars

- Cane sugar
- Honey
- Maple syrup
- High fructose corn syrup
- Agave nectar
- Turbinado sugar

Sugar-Alcohols

- Maltitol
- Xylitol

- Sorbitol (found in chewing gum)

Packaged/Processed Foods

- Margarine
- MSG (Mono Sodium Glutamate)
- Ice creams
- Wheat gluten
- Fast food
- Candies
- Baked goods like cakes and cookies
- Sodas/soft drinks
- Almond milk products
- Dried fruits
- Gelatin

Artificial Sweeteners

- Saccharin
- Splenda
- Equal
- Aspartame
- Sucralose
- Acesulfame

Over 30 Delicious Foods You can eat

Healthy Animal Fats

- Ghee
- Lard
- Grass-fed butter
- Cream cheese
- Egg yolks
- Tallow
- Organ meat e.g. bone marrow, liver, tongue
- Shellfish e.g. lobster, crab, scallops, squid, shrimp, prawns
- Wild-caught fish e.g. salmon, mackerel, snapper, halibut, tuna, cod, trout, eel

Cooking Oils

- Unrefined coconut oil
- Avocado oil
- Olive oil

Nuts and Seeds

- Walnuts
- Pine nuts
- Pistachios
- Pecans
- Cashews
- Hazelnuts
- Sunflower seeds
- Hemp seeds
- Chia seeds
- Sesame seeds
- Flax oil
- Macadamia oil
- Walnut oil

Vegetables

- Celery
- Tomatoes
- Kale
- Brussels sprouts
- Bok Choy
- Onion
- Garlic
- Peppers
- Eggplant
- Cucumber
- Fresh herbs (e.g. cilantro, chives, mint, rosemary, parsley, basil)
- Mushrooms
- Lettuce
- Zucchini
- Endive
- Fennel
- Radicchio

Animal Protein

- Pork
- Chicken
- Beef
- Wild game
- Turkey

- Duck
- Bone Broth

Fruit

- Strawberries
- Blackberries
- Blueberries

Others/Supplements

- Spirulina
- Mustard
- Mayonnaise
- Sauerkraut
- Allspice
- Pesto
- Dark organic chocolate
- MCT oil
- Almond flour
- Unsweetened nut milk e.g. coconut milk, hazelnut milk, cashew milk, hemp milk, almond milk)
- Omega-3
- Magnesium
- Sodium
- Glutamine
- Taurine

- Raspberries
- Apple
- Lime
- Lemon
- Pears

- Chlorella
- Fish oil supplements
- Maca Root
- Raw cacao powder
- Coconut flour
- Herbal coffee and tea (with no sugar)
- Mineral water or Seltzer

- BCAAs (Branch Chain Amino Acids)
- Whey protein
- Essential amino acid

Yummy Breakfast Recipes to Start Your Morning Right

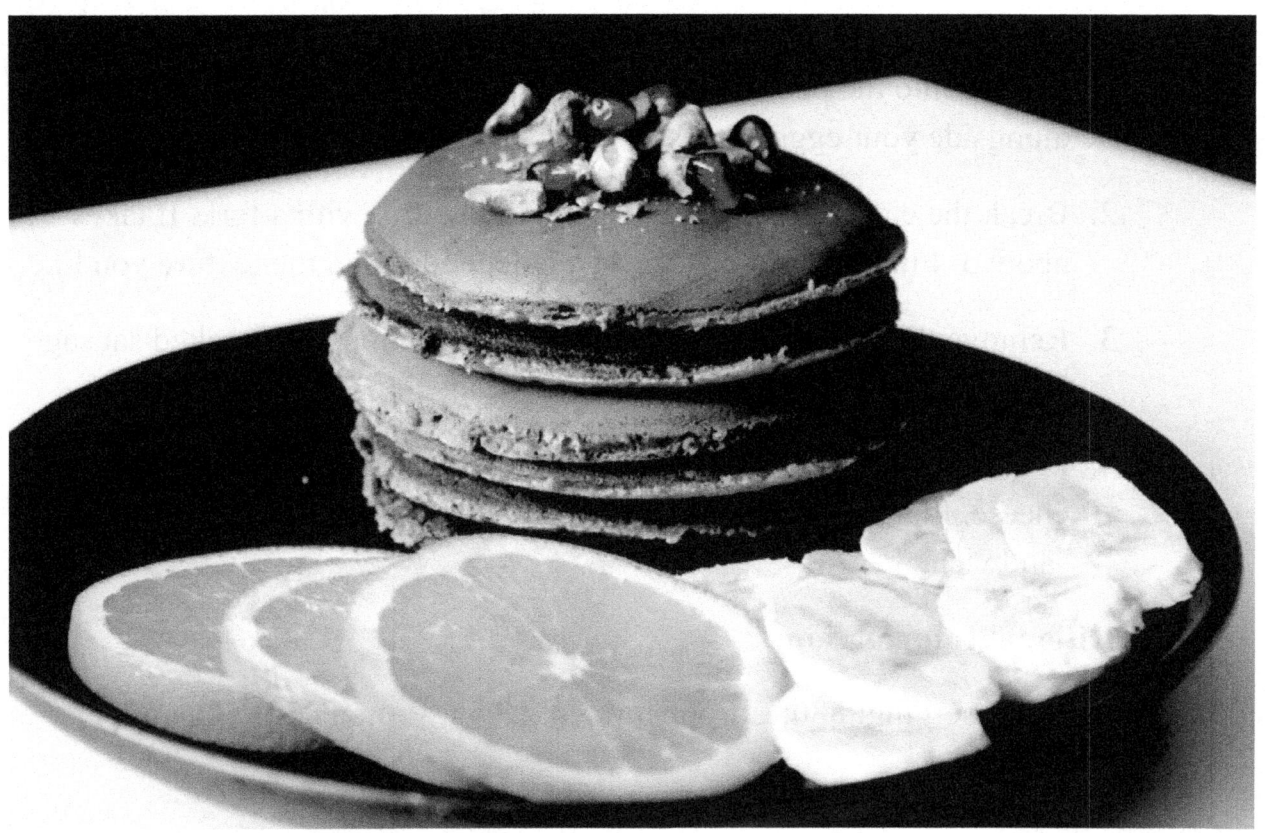

Sausage and Egg Muffin

(Total time: 10 min | Serves: 1)

Ingredients:

- 2 Large Eggs
- 1 tbsp. butter
- 1 tbsp. mayonnaise
- 2 sausages
- 2 slices cheddar cheese

- Slices of avocado

Instructions:

1. In a large pan, heat the butter at a medium temperature and put the moulds into the pan. If you can't get pre-cooked patties, just fry them alongside your eggs.

2. Break the eggs into the moulds and gently mix with a fork. It takes about 3-4 minutes to cook the eggs, depending on the texture you like.

3. Remove the eggs. Take one, and add half the mayo, a cooked sausage patty, then half the cheese and the avocado.

4. Put the second sausage on top of the avocado, finish off with the cheese. Put the remaining mayo on the other egg, and complete the sandwich.

Nutritional Information:

Calories per serving: 880; Carbohydrates: 10.5g; Protein: 32g; Fat: 82g.

Breakfast Loaf with Berry and Peanut Butter

(Total time: 1hr.| Serves: 6)

Ingredients:

- ½ c. peanut butter
- ¼ c. melted butter
- 5 eggs
- ½ c. milk
- 1 tsp. vanilla extract
- ½ c. almond flour
- 3 tbsps. sweetener
- 2 tsps. baking powder
- ½ tsp. sea salt
- ½ c. mixed berries

Instructions:

1. Heat the oven to 350 degrees. Either use a silicon loaf pan, or use an ordinary loaf pan lined with grease-proof parchment paper.

2. Combine the peanut butter, melted butter and eggs in a large bowl. Mix until thoroughly combined.

3. Add the milk and vanilla extract, and mix.

4. Using a different bowl, mix together the flour, baking powder, sea salt and sweetener. Make sure that they are thoroughly combined.

5. Mix the contents of the first bowl into the second, stirring all the time.

6. Use a spatula to carefully fold the berries into the mixture.

7. Pour the contents into the loaf tin, and bake for approximately 45 minutes.

8. After 45 minutes use a toothpick or fine knife to check it is cooked, (the toothpick should come out clean). If necessary, cook for up to 15 more minutes, checking every five minutes.

9. Toast or eat fresh with butter.

Nutritional Information:

Calories per serving: 150; Carbohydrates: 5g; Protein: 6g; Fat: 15g.

Keto Cereal

(Total time: 15 mins.| Serves: 3)

Ingredients:

- 1½ c. shredded coconut
- Sweetener
- Sea salt
- ½ tsp. cinnamon
- 1 c. toasted walnut
- 1 c. toasted macadamia pieces
- 1 c. toasted flax seeds
- Milk

Instructions:

1. Simply combine the ingredients.
2. If desired, the contents can be heated gently.
3. Serve with almond milk if desired.

Nutritional Information:

Calories per serving: 350; Carbohydrates: 2g; Protein: 22g; Fat: 24g.

Ham and Cheese Waffles

(Total time: 20 mins.| Serves: 2)

Ingredients:

- 2 oz. Chopped ham steak
- 2 oz. Grated cheddar cheese
- Dried basil
- Paprika
- 1 tsp. Baking powder
- 8 eggs
- 3 scoops of protein powder
- 12 tbsps. Melted butter
- 1 tsp. Salt

Instructions:

1. Separate 4 of the eggs into two bowls (separate yolk from whites) set the other 4 eggs aside.
2. Add the powder, baking powder, butter and sea salt to the yolks and whisk together.
3. Fold in the cheese and ham.
4. Whisk the egg whites together with the salt either with hand beaters or in the mixer until stiff.
5. Gently fold half of the whites into the egg yolk mixture. Leave for a few moments, then fold in the remaining egg white.
6. Add around a quarter of a cup of the mixture to a waffle maker, per waffle to be cooked. Cook for about four minutes until lightly browned.
7. Store in the fridge or freeze.
8. Heat the waffles in the toaster and while they're toasting, fry an egg on the stove top.
9. Serve an egg on the waffle, and top with paprika and basil.

Nutritional Information:

Calories per serving: 620; Carbohydrates: 1g; Protein: 45g; Fat: 50g.

Baked Eggs with Avocado

(Total time: 20 mins.| Serves: 4)

Ingredients:

- 2 medium avocado
- 4 medium eggs
- ¼ tsp. garlic powder
- ¼ tsp. sea salt
- ¼ tsp. black pepper
- A handful of grated Parmesan cheese

Instructions:

1. Preheat the oven to 350 degrees.

2. Cut the avocado in half, remove the stone and scoop out about a quarter of the flesh from each half. This is to create enough space for the egg.

3. Put the avocado halves in something to keep them stable, like a muffin tin.

4. Sprinkle the two halves with the sea salt, the black pepper and the garlic powder.

5. Crack the eggs so that one fits into each half. Sprinkle with the cheese.

6. Bake for about 15 minutes, or until the whites are set and are firm if the pan is shaken.

Nutritional Information:

Calories per serving: 261; Carbohydrates: 3g; Protein: 14g; Fat: 20g.

Cheese, Egg and Bacon Cups

(Total time: 20 mins.| Serves: 6)

Ingredients:

- 6 bacon strips
- 6 large eggs
- A handful of spinach
- ¼ c. cheese
- Salt
- pepper

Instructions:

1. Preheat the oven to 400 degrees.
2. Fry up the bacon, and set aside to cool and drain. This could be prepped in advance.
3. Grease a muffin tin with oil, and line with a slice of bacon. Press the bacon down so the ends will stick up, these will become the handles with which you remove the cups later.
4. Beat the eggs in a bowl.
5. Drain and pat dry the spinach in some paper towels. Chop roughly (this can be prepped in advance) and add to the eggs.
6. Put about a quarter of the cup of the mixture into each muffin place, so that they fill it up to the three-quarter mark.
7. Sprinkle with cheese, and season to taste
8. Bake in the middle of the oven for about 15 minutes.
9. You can even freeze these and microwave for breakfast if desired.

Nutritional Information:

Calories per serving: 101; Carbohydrates: 1g; Protein: 8g; Fat: 7g.

Yoghurt Parfait

(Total time: 10 mins.| Serves: 4)

Ingredients:

- 2 c. natural, full fat yoghurt
- 1 c. shredded coconut
- Sweetener.
- 1 c. toasted walnut pieces
- 1 c. toasted macadamia pieces

- 1 c. toasted flax seeds
- 4 sliced bananas
- 4 Handfuls of sliced strawberries
- 4 Handfuls of sliced blueberries

Instructions:

1. Take a glass serving jar, such as a Sundae dish or mug.

2. Place three tbsp. of the yoghurt in the bottom of the container.

3. Add sweetener if desired.

4. Add a layer of nuts.

5. Add a layer of the coconut.

6. Add the banana.

7. Alternate layers of fruit and nuts.

8. Pour the remaining yoghurt on top.

Nutritional Information:

Calories per serving: 230; Carbohydrates: 9g; Protein: 20g; Fat: 15g.

Salad with chicken breast and spinach

(Total time: 55 mins.| Serves: 3)

Ingredients:

- 3.5 oz. chicken breast
- 2 tbsps. spinach
- 1¾ oz. lettuce
- 1 bell pepper;
- 2 tbsps. olive oil
- 1 tbsp. lemon juice

Instructions:

1. Boil the chicken breast without adding salt, and then cut it into small strips.

2. Put the spinach in boiling water for a few minutes, then cut it into small strips.

3. Cut the pepper in strips as well.

4. Mix all the ingredients, add oil and juice.

Nutrition information:

Calories per serving: 100, Fat: 11g, Carbohydrates: 3g, Protein: 6g

Bacon lemon thyme breakfast muffins

(Total time: 35 mins.| Serves: 6)

Ingredients:

- 3 c. almond flour
- 1 c. bacon.
- ½ c. melted ghee
- 4 eggs
- 2 tsps. lemon thyme
- 1 tsp. baking soda
- 1 tsp. salt.

Instructions:

- Set your oven to 350° F.
- Use a mixing bowl to melt ghee.
- Add the eggs, almond flour, lemon thyme, baking soda, and salt.
- Mix everything well.
- Add the bacon bits.
- Line muffin liners on a muffin pan.
- Pour the mixture into the muffin pan (to around ¾ full).
- Bake for 19 minutes.

Nutrition Information:

Calories per serving: 300, Fat: 28g, Carbohydrates: 7g, Protein: 11g

Cheese omelet with bacon

(Total time: 20 mins.| Serves: 1)

Ingredients:

- 3 eggs
- 5 slices bacon
- 1 tbsp. ghee
- Sea salt
- Chili pepper

Instructions:

1. Cut the bacon strips into pieces and fry them over the high heat.

2. Whisk eggs with salt and pepper in a bowl.

3. Pour the mixture into a frying pan with the bacon, cover with a lid, and fry over low heat for about 10 minutes.

4. Check occasionally for doneness.

Nutritional Information:

Calories per serving: 420, Protein: 24g, Fat: 35g, Carbohydrates: 2g

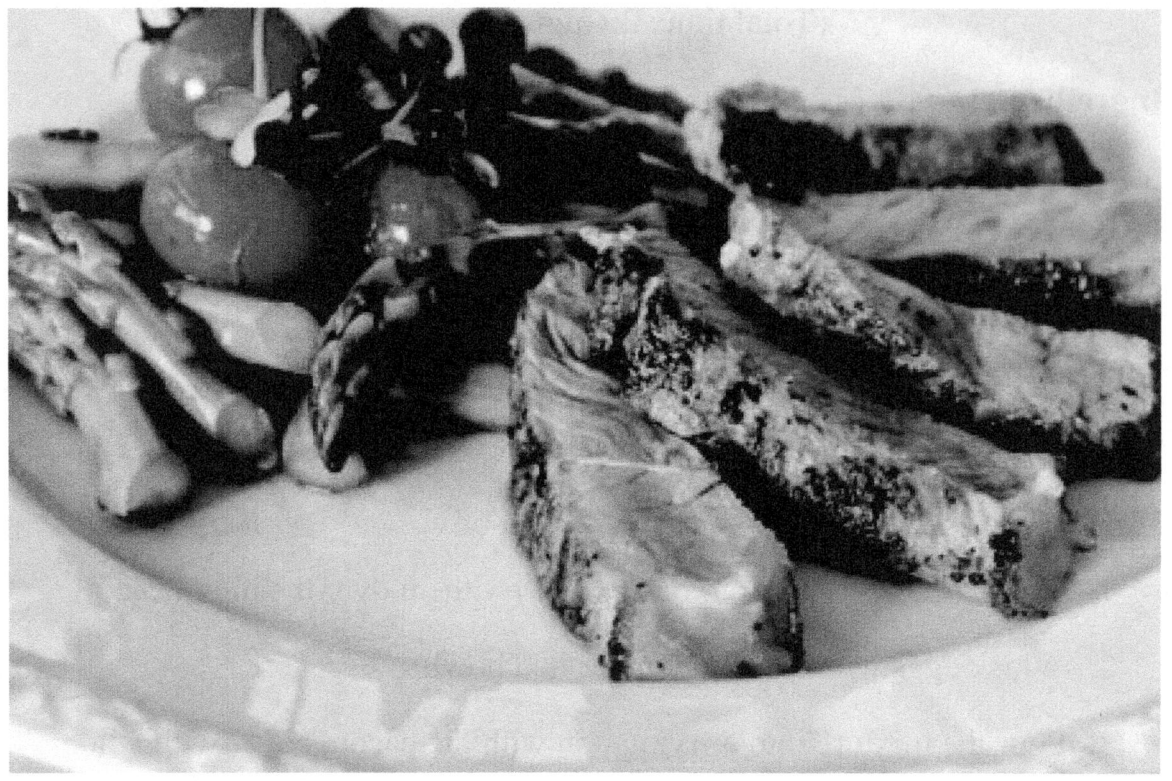

Buffalo Chicken Lettuce Wraps

(Total time: 15 mins.| Serves: 4)

Ingredients:

- ½ red pepper
- ½ green pepper
- 4 stalks of celery
- 2 lbs. chicken thighs
- 2 chopped scallions
- ½ c. crumbled blue cheese

- 2 tsps. onion powder
- 1 tsp. garlic powder
- 2 tbsps. butter
- Salt
- pepper
- Hot sauce
- 8 large lettuce leaves

Instructions:

1. Melt the butter in a large pan.
2. Add the peppers and celery and sauté for about five minutes
3. Add the chick, onion and garlic. Stir and season. Cook for about five minutes until the chicken is cooked.
4. Add the hot sauce (if using), stir and heat for another minute.
5. Remove the pan from the heat, and add the cheese and scallions, stirring all the time.
6. Put three tablespoons of the mixture into a lettuce leaf and enjoy.

Nutritional Information:

Calories per serving: 547; Carbohydrates: 3g; Protein: 50g; Fat: 37g.

Vegetarian Cauliflower Curry

(Total time: 55 mins.| Serves: 6)

Ingredients:

For the Main Dish:

- 1 head of cauliflower
- 1½ c. of full fat yoghurt
- 2 tbsps. curry powder
- 1 tsp. paprika
- 1 tsp. cayenne pepper
- 1 lime
- 1 tsp. salt
- ½ tsp. black pepper
- 2 tsps. lime zest

For the Topping:

- ¼ c. sun dried tomatoes
- ½ c. pine nuts
- 1 tbsp. cilantro
- 2 tbsps. feta cheese
- ¼ c. olive oil
- A clove of garlic

Instructions:

1. Warm the oven to 375 degrees, and take a baking sheet lines with grease proof paper, or parchment paper.

2. In a large bowl, take all the main ingredients (not those for the topping) except the cauliflower. Mix them together then rub it all over the outside of the cauliflower head.

3. Cook for 45 minutes until the cauliflower is crispy and a lovely golden color. Let it cool.

4. Make the topping. Put the garlic, sun dried tomatoes and half of the pine nuts into a blender and blast until chunky.

5. Add the rest of the ingredients for the topping and mix carefully.

6. Carefully cut the heads from the main cauliflower and place in shallow dish.

7. Drizzle the topping over the cauliflower and warm gently.

Nutritional Information:

Calories per serving: 260; Carbohydrates: 7g; Protein: 10g; Fat: 20g.

Beef Burritos

(Total time: 8 hrs.| Serves: 4)

Ingredients:

For the Beef:

- 2 lbs. sirloin steak
- 1 c. chicken broth
- 1 c. BBQ sauce
- ½ onion
- 2 tsps. salt
- ½ tsp. black pepper
- 5 fresh cloves of garlic
- ½ tsp. cinnamon
- 2 bay leaves
- For the Taco
- 8 low carb wraps
- ½ c. mayo
- 1½ c. coleslaw

Instructions:

1. Pat dry the sirloin with paper towels, and score along the sides.
2. Combine the salt, pepper and cinnamon. Sprinkle it evenly onto the steak, making sure that there is an even covering.
3. Put the onion and garlic in the slow cooker. Place the beef on top and cover with the soup. Add the bay leaves and cook for eight hours.
4. When cooked, remove and strain the ingredients. Then shred the beef mix by pulling it with two forks.
5. Add the BBQ sauce and combine everything well.
6. Put some of the beef into the wrap, add coleslaw and dash of mayo. Wrap and eat.

Nutritional Information:

Calories per serving: 750, Carbohydrates: 14g; Protein: 60g; Fat: 50g

Open-Faced Prosciutto and Brie Sandwich with Avocado Bun

(Total time: 20 mins.| Serves: 2)

Ingredients:

- 1 avocado
- 4 small slices of brie
- 8 thin slices of prosciutto
- 6 mushrooms
- 2 c. raw spinach

- 2 tsps. butter
- 1 tsp. sesame seeds
- ½ tsp. salt
- ¼ tsp. black pepper

Instructions:

1. Cook the spinach for five minutes until it has wilted. Drain and squeeze out excess water.

2. Slice the mushroom and sauté in the butter until soft. Add some pepper and salt.

3. Cut the avocado in half. Do this by cutting until the pit is reached, then rotating and twisting until the avocado splits. Remove the stone and scoop out the flesh. Cut a slice off the bottom of one half of the avocado so it can stand. This will be your 'bottom slice of bread'.

4. Fill the two halves of your avocado with the ingredients. Serve as open-faced sandwich

Nutritional Information:

Calories per serving: 482, Carbohydrates: 12g; Protein: 16g; Fat: 40g.

Keto Cubano

(Total time: 15 mins.| Serves: 4)

Ingredients:

- Thinly sliced dill pickles
- 1/3 lb. sliced cooked ham
- 1/3 lb. cooked pork tenderloin
- ¼ lb. sliced Swiss cheese
- 1 tbsp. melted butter
- 2 tbsps. mayonnaise
- 2 tbsps. Dijon mustard
- Low Carb wraps OR bib lettuce

Instructions:

1. Mix the mustard and mayo together and spread over the wrap (if using low carb wrap)

2. Divide up the pickle, cheese and meats between the sandwiches. Roll up the wraps tightly

3. Place in a sandwich maker, or in a panini press and cook for five to seven minutes.

4. If using the lettuce instead of the wraps, simply omit step 3.

Nutritional Information:

Calories per serving: 472, Carbohydrates: 7g; Protein: 28g; Fat: 36g.

Keto Monkey Bread

(Total time: 30 mins.| Serves: 3)

Ingredients:

- 2 baby eggplants
- ¾ c. mozzarella cheese
- 2 tbsps. melted butter
- 1 tbsp. fresh basil
- 1 clove of garlic

Instructions:

1. Heat the oven to 375 degrees.

2. Take a muffin pan and lightly grease.

3. Combine the garlic, melted butter and a half of the basil.

4. Place some of the eggplant (four or five pieces) into the bottom of each muffin tray.

5. Sprinkle even amounts of mozzarella and drizzle butter mixture over each portion of eggplant

6. Add the remaining cheese on top and bake for around twenty minutes. The cheese should be nicely browned.

7. Allow to cool for five minutes and eat warm; you can reheat later.

Nutritional Information:

Calories per serving: 195, Carbohydrates: 6g; Protein: 8g; Fat: 15g.

Cauliflower Grits With Roasted Mushrooms And Walnuts

(Total time: 30 mins.| Serves: 4)

Ingredients:

- 6 sliced mushrooms
- 3 garlic cloves
- ½ c. walnuts
- ½ c. water
- 1 c. half-and-half
- 1 c. grated cheddar
- 2 tbsps. butter
- 600g cauliflower
- 2 tbsps. olive oil
- 1 tbsp. fresh rosemary
- 1 tbsp. smoked paprika
- ¼ tsp. salt

Instructions:

1. Heat the oven to 400 degrees F and line a baking tray with foil.

2. Combine the garlic, rosemary, walnuts, paprika and mushrooms with a touch of salt, and drizzle with oil.

3. Roast on the tray for fifteen minutes.

4. Cut and pulse the cauliflower heads in a processor until very fine, like rice.

5. Steam the cauliflower in a pot with a half cup of water. Do this for about five minutes as you want it tender, but not soft.

6. Pour in the half-and-half and simmer for three minutes.

7. Add the cheese and butter, and stir on a low heat. If the resulting mixture is not runny enough for your taste, add another half cup of water.

8. Add the hot mushroom and walnut mix to the top of the grits and eat warm.

Nutritional Information:

Calories per serving: 452, Carbohydrates: 11g; Protein: 16g; Fat: 36g.

Spicy Roast Beef Cups

(Total time: 20 mins.| Serves: 1)

Ingredients:

- 6 thin slices of deli counter cooked roast beef
- 1 tbsp. sour cream
- 1½ tbsps. hot chili
- ½ c. grated cheddar cheese

Instructions:

1. Break the beef up into small chunks, and layer half in the bottom of your cup, dish or mug.

2. Cover the beef with the cream sour, spreading it out.

3. Add a third of the chili

4. Spread a third of the cheese

5. Repeat numbers one to four.

6. Top with the remaining cheese and chili.

7. Microwave for some minutes to melt the cheese.

Nutritional Information:

Calories per serving: 270, Carbohydrates: 4g; Protein: 23g; Fat: 18g.

Crispy Pork Salad

(Total time: 50 mins.| Serves: 2)

Ingredients:

- ½ lb. pork belly slices
- 1/3 c. blue cheese
- ¼ pear
- 2 c. salad leaves
- 2 tsps. salt
- 1/3 c. chopped walnuts
- 1 tbsp. of stevia
- 1 tsp. water
- ½ tsp. Dijon mustard
- ½ tsp. any whole grain mustard for the dressing
- 2 tbsp. of white wine vinegar
- 2 tsp. olive oil

Instructions:

1. Cover the pork with half of the olive oil. Cook in a hot oven until crunchy and browned, about 20 to 30 minutes.

2. Warm a pan and add the water and stevia to the pan, and add the walnuts once the stevia has dissolved. Cook for five minutes until the liquid has caramelised the walnuts.

3. Tip the nuts onto a tray and leave to cool. Note: they will be hot.

4. Chop the pear and cheese into bite-sized pieces.

5. Make the vinaigrette by adding the mustards, vinegar and oil into a bowl and mixing well.

6. By this time the pork should be cooked. Remove set aside to cool, then chop into bite sized chunks.

7. Toss the salad in the vinaigrette and add the pork, nuts, cheese and pear.

Nutritional Information:

Calories per serving: 1050, Carbohydrates: 5g; Protein: 13g; Fat: 55g.

Goat Cheese and Vegetable Salad

(Total time: 30 mins.| Serves: 2)

Ingredients:

- 4 rounds of goat cheese
- 1 red pepper
- 4 c. water cress
- 1 tbsp. oil

- ¼ c. sliced button mushrooms
- 1 tsp. chopped onion
- 1 tsp. chopped garlic
- 4 tbsp. Sesame see

Instructions:

1. Combine the seeds, onion and garlic in a dish.

2. Coat each piece of goat cheese in the mix, lightly coating both sides. Refrigerate.

3. Char the peppers and mushrooms in a pan with a spray of oil. Don't overcook, heat until the pepper starts to soften and darken.

4. Put the watercress into two bowls and add the pepper and mushroom to the top.

5. Fry the goat cheese on both sides, for about thirty seconds on each side. Take care flipping, as the cheese will already be starting to melt.

6. Add to the bowls, and drizzle with the oil.

Nutritional Information:

Calories per serving: 350, Carbohydrates: 7g; Protein: 16g; Fat: 28g.

Dinner Is Never Boring with These Water-Mouthing Meals

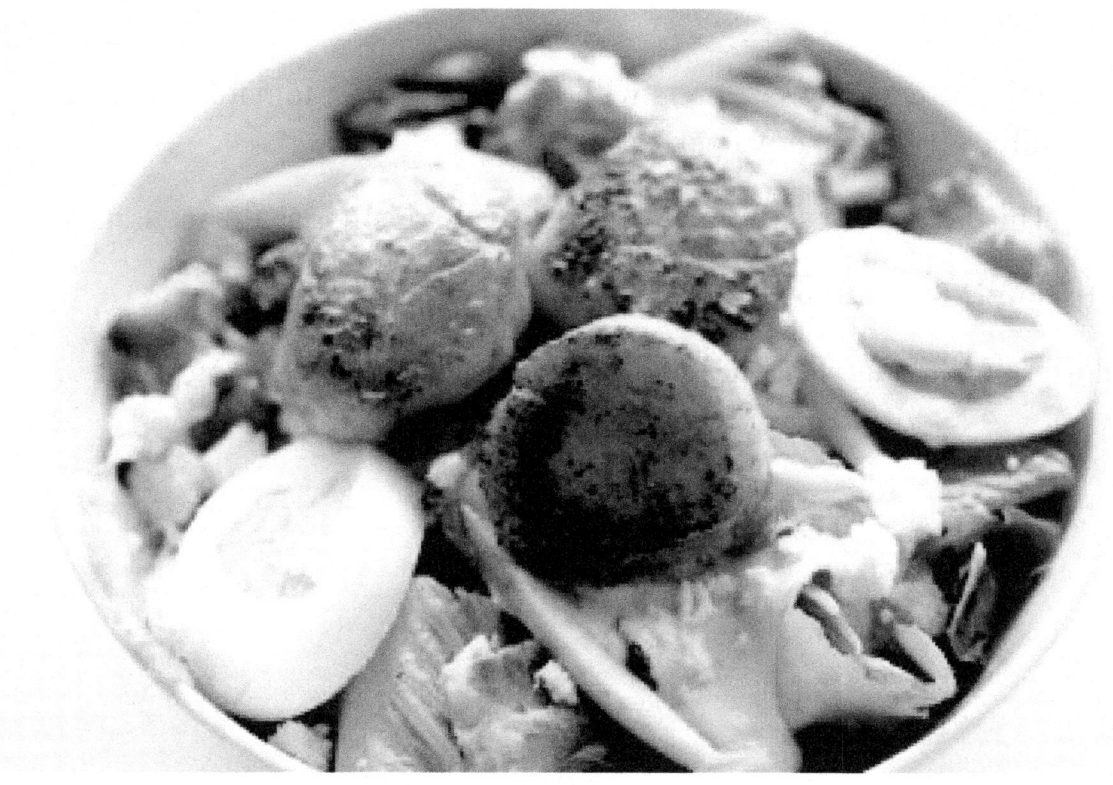

Cauliflower Taboule Salad

(Total time: 15 mins.| Serves: 1)

Ingredients:

- 3 oz. Cauliflower florets
- 2 tbsps. Parsley
- 6 mint leaves
- 2 diced tomatoes
- 2 cucumbers

- 6 tbsps. Lemon juice
- 2 tbsps. Olive oil
- Salt
- Pepper

Instructions:

1. Make a couscous-like mass from the cauliflower florets by mincing them.

2. Mix the cauliflower florets with finely cut herbs, tomatoes, lemon, olive oil, salt, and pepper.

3. This tasty fresh salad may be used as a garnish or as the meal itself.

Nutrition Information:

Calories per serving: 80, Carbohydrates: 6g, Protein: 2g, Fat: 6g

Thai Chicken with cauliflower rice

(Total time: 15 mins.| Serves: 3)

Ingredients:

- 1 cauliflower head
- 1 tbsp. ginger
- 3 eggs
- 3 chilies
- 3 cloves of garlic

- 4 cooked chicken breasts, shredded
- Salt
- Coconut oil
- 1 tbsp. tamari soy sauce
- ½ c. chopped parsley

Instructions:

1. Break the cauliflower into florets and process in a blender until it forms a rice-like texture.

2. Put the cauliflower into a large pan with the coconut oil and cook the cauliflower rice, stirring, on medium heat until it is soft.

3. In a separate pan, scramble the eggs with some coconut oil.

4. The next step is to add scrambled eggs to cauliflower rice. Add the ginger, garlic, and the chopped chilies.

5. When the cauliflower rice mixture is soft, add the shredded chicken meat.

6. Add the tamari soy sauce and salt to taste.

7. Mix well. Garnish with fresh coriander or parsley.

Nutrition Information:

Calories per serving: 350, Fat: 11g, Carbohydrates: 9g, Protein: 55g

Spinach salad with bacon and blue cheese

(Total time: 20 mins.| Serves: 1)

Ingredients:

- 2½ oz. spinach

- 1 red onion

- 4 tbsps. blue cheese

- 2 oz. almond

- 5 oz. bacon strips.

Instructions:

1. Fry the bacon strips on each side for 2-3 minutes. You don't need to add any oil because the bacon's fat is enough.

2. Cut the bacon. For serving you need a salad plate.

3. Place the spinach leaves on the bottom, then the sliced onion, cheese, and bacon.

4. Top it up with the almond nibs.

5. Use salad dressing if you like. This salad differs from the other green salads because of the blue cheese taste. It is an excellent low-carb salad.

Nutritional Information:

Calories per serving: 420, Protein: 24g, Fat: 35g, Carbohydrates: 2g

Grilled chicken skewers with garlic sauce

(Total time: 20 mins.| Serves: 2)

Ingredients:

- 8 oz. chicken breast,

- 2 small onions

- 2 bell peppers, chopped;

- 1 zucchini.

For the Garlic Sauce:

- 7 cloves of garlic

- 1 tsp. salt;

- ¼ c. lemon juice;

- 1 c. olive oil.

- Additional ingredients for the marinade: ½ cup olive oil;

- 1 tsp. salt.

Instructions:

1. Heat the grill to high. Soak wooden skewers in water first. For the garlic sauce, put the garlic cloves and salt into the blender.

2. Add ⅛ cup of the lemon juice and ½ cup of olive oil. Blend well for 5-10 seconds.

3. Keep half the garlic sauce for serving.

4. Take the other half of the garlic sauce and add the ½ cup of olive oil and salt. Mix well.

5. Chop the onions, bell peppers, and zucchini into approximately 1-inch cubes or squares. Put them into the garlic marinade.

6. Thread the vegetable and chicken cubes onto the soaked skewers and grill on high until the chicken cooked. Serve with the reserved garlic sauce.

Nutrition Information:

Calories per servings: 580, Fat: 33g, Carbohydrates: 11g, Protein: 55g

Pasta with chicken and basil

(Total time: 30 mins.| Serves: 1)

Ingredients:

- 2 chicken fillets
- 2 tbsps. Ghee
- 1 lb. Diced tomatoes
- ½ c. Basil
- ¼ c. Coconut milk
- 1 clove of garlic
- Salt;
- 1 shredded zucchini

Instructions:

1. Sauté cubed chicken in ghee until done.

2. Add tomatoes and salt. Simmer and reduce the liquid. Meanwhile, do the preparation for the pasta.

3. Shred zucchini in a food processor if you have one.

4. Mix the garlic, coconut milk, basil, chicken, garlic and coconut milk and cook for some more time.

5. Using a bowl, put half of pasta, top with the creamy chicken.

Nutrition Info:

Calories per serving: 540, Fat: 27g, Carbohydrates: 13g, Protein: 59g

Salmon Fishcakes

(Total time: 20 mins.| Serves: 2)

Ingredients:

- 2 large eggs
- 4 ounces sliced smoked salmon
- ½ tbsp. butter
- 2 tbsp. fresh chives
- Salt and Pepper
- Jar of ready-made Hollandaise sauce

Instructions:

1. Boil the eggs for ten to twelve minutes. They need to be hard boiled.
2. Dice the salmon finely while the eggs are cooking.
3. Heat the butter under a high heat. Put half the salmon in to crisp it up, then set aside.
4. Run the eggs under cold water and peel.
5. Mash the eggs using a fork until they are broken up into fine pieces.
6. Take the raw salmon and half of the chives and mix with the egg and two to three tbsp. of Hollandaise sauce.
7. Split the mixture into four lumps and form into rough balls.
8. Mix the crispy salmon and remaining chives together and dip the egg balls into them until fully coated.

Nutritional Information:

Calories per serving: 295, Fat: 23g, Carbohydrates: 1g, Protein: 18g

Baby back Ribs

(Total time: 1 hr.| Serves: 5)

Ingredients:

For the Ribs

- A rack of baby back ribs
- 1 c. water
- ¼ c. apple cider vinegar
- 2 tsps. liquid smoke
- 1 tbsp. paprika
- ½ tbsp. crushed garlic
- ½ tbsp. diced onion
- ½ tsp. black pepper
- ½ tbsp. chili powder
- ½ tbsp. cumin
- ½ tsp. cayenne pepper
- ½ tsp. mustard powder
- 1 tsp. salt

For the BBQ sauce

- 1½ c. mayo
- ¼ c. apple cider vinegar
- 1 tbsp. Dijon mustard

- 1 tsp. black pepper

- 1 tsp. salt

- 1 tsp. crushed garlic

- 2 tbsps. sweetener

- 2 tsps. ready-made horseradish sauce

Instructions:

1. Put the paprika, the half tablespoon of crushed garlic, onion, half a tsp of black pepper, the chili powder, cumin, cayenne pepper, mustard powder and a tsp of salt in a bowl and combine.

2. Rinse the ribs in water and pat dry.

3. Remove the skin from the back of the ribs. To do this, place the tip of a sharp knife under the end of the skin and work the skin free, then pull carefully and it should all come away.

4. Rub the spice into the meat making sure it is fully covered.

5. Add the ribs, quarter cup of apple cider vinegar, water and liquid smoke to the put.

6. Seal the pot and cook on high for 35 minutes, allowing the steam to naturally release.

7. Meanwhile, whisk together all the remaining ingredients to make the sauce. Store the sauce in the fridge for at least two hours to allow the sauce to develop its flavor.

8. Preheat the grill to 450 degrees, and grill the ribs for about six minutes on each side.

9. Serve with the sauce.

Nutritional Information:

Calories per serving: 650, Fat: 42g, Carbohydrates: 3g, Protein: 57g

Garlic Cream Pork Chops

(Total time: 30 mins.| Serves: 4)

Ingredients:

- 4 boneless pork chops
- 1 tbsp. paprika
- 1 tsp. crushed garlic
- ¾ chopped onion
- 1 tsp. black pepper
- 1 tsp. salt
- ¼ tsp. cayenne pepper
- 2 tbsps. coconut oil
- 1 c. sliced mushrooms
- 1 tbsp. butter
- ½ c. heavy cream
- 1 tbsp. parsley, freshly chopped

Instructions:

1. Mix together the paprika, garlic, one third of the onion you have prepared, salt, pepper and cayenne pepper. Sprinkle onto both sides of the chops and rub in.

2. Heat the coconut oil and brown the chops, about three minutes per side.

3. Take the chops and leave to one side.

4. In the pan, add the rest of the onions and the mushroom and cook for three or four minutes, until the onions go clear.

5. In a separate pan whisk the cream and butter under a low heat.

6. Put the chops and cream sauce back in the pan and cook for about five minutes in each side, making sure that the cream is stirred regularly.

Nutritional Information:

Calories per serving: 481, Fat: 32g, Carbohydrates: 4g, Protein: 15g

Spaghetti Carbonara

(Total time: 30 mins.| Serves: 4)

Ingredients:

- 1½ tbsps. butter
- 5 oz. chopped thick cut bacon
- 3 packets shirataki noodles
- 3 large eggs
- 1 c. grated Parmesan cheese
- 2 large minced cloves garlic

Instructions:

1. Melt butter in a large pan.

2. Cook the bacon until crispy.

3. Add the garlic, then the noodles.

4. Stir the noodles, as they heat.

5. While the noodles are heating, in a different bowl, beat the eggs and three quarters of the cheese.

6. When the noodles are fully heated, pop them into another bowl.

7. Stir the egg and cheese mixture while the noodles are still warm. The sauce should thicken to a thick consistency, but not solidify.

8. Top with parsley and the rest of the cheese.

Nutritional Information:

Calories per serving: 361, Fat: 29g, Carbohydrates: 4.5g, Protein: 16g

Shrimp in Tuscan Cream Sauce

(Total time: 30 mins.| Serves: 4)

Ingredients:

- 1 lb. raw shrimp
- 1 tbsp. butter
- 1 c. cubed cream cheese
- ½ c. whole milk
- 2 cloves garlic
- 1 tsp. dried basil
- 1 tsp. salt
- ½ c. Parmesan
- 5 sun-dried tomatoes
- ¼ c. baby kale

Instructions:

1. Melt the butter in a large pan.
2. Add the shrimp and lower the temperature.
3. Cook the shrimp for thirty seconds, then turn them and cook until they are beginning to turn pink.
4. Add the cream cheese.
5. Pour milk into the pan and increase the heat. Stir until the cheese has melted and there are no lumps.
6. Add the garlic, salt and basil and continue stirring.
7. Throw in the cheese, and finish stirring once it has melted in. Leave the dish to simmer until the sauce shows signs of thickening.
8. Finally add the tomatoes and kale.
9. Serve straight away.

Nutritional Information:

Calories per serving: 298, Fat: 18, Carbohydrates: 6.5g, Protein: 23g

Delightful Snacks Meals

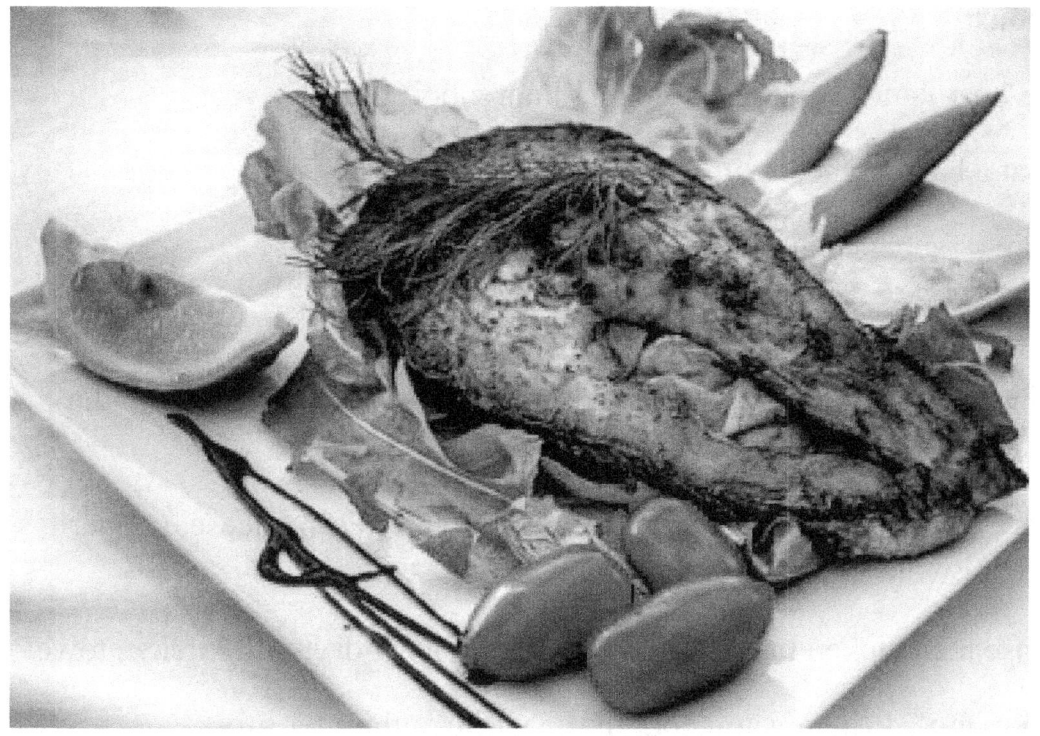

Herb Dressed Chicken Parmesan Fingers

(Total time: 45 mins.| Serves: 6)

Ingredients:

- 2 lbs. boneless chicken breast
- 4 garlic cloves
- 4 oz. butter
- 1 c. grated parmesan cheese
- 2 tbsps. chopped thyme
- 1 tsp. chili pepper flakes
- Sea salt

- Black pepper

Instructions:

1. Pre-heat your oven to 350-degree Fahrenheit

2. Coat a baking sheet with non-stick cooking spray

3. Take a saucepan and place it over medium-heat

4. Add butter and melt the butter, swirl to coat well

5. Stir in garlic and Sauté until fragrant, remove the heat and keep the garlic on the side for 15 minutes

6. Take a bowl and add thyme, chili pepper, parmesan cheese, pepper and stir well

7. Rinse the chicken breast thoroughly and blot it dry with kitchen towel

8. Slice into 24 fingers and coat in the garlic and butter mix

9. Dredge the fingers in the cheese mix and arrange them on your baking sheet

10. Bake for 25-30 minutes until the fingers are golden brown

11. Transfer them to a cooling rack and allow them to cool

Nutritional Information:

Calories per serving: 370, Fat: 20g, Carbohydrates: 6g, Protein: 40g

Bacon Moza Sticks

(Total time: 15 mins.| Serves: 4)

Ingredients:

- 8 bacon strips
- 4 mozzarella string cheese pieces
- Sunflower oil

Instructions:

1. Take a heavy-duty skillet over medium heat and add about 2 inches of oil
2. Heat it up to 350-degree Fahrenheit
3. Have each string cheese to 8 pieces
4. Wrap each piece of string cheese with strip of bacon and secure using toothpick
5. Cook the sticks in oil for 2 minutes until the bacon is browned
6. Place the sticks on plate lined with kitchen towel and drain
7. Serve!

Nutritional Information:

Calories per serving: 278, Fat: 15, Carbohydrates: 3g, Protein: 32g

Buffalo Chicken Dip

(Total time: 30 mins.| Serves: 4)

Ingredients:

- 6 whole eggs
- Water
- 6 oz. cooked chicken
- 3 tbsps. mayonnaise
- 1½ tbsps. red buffalo wing sauce
- ¼ c. blue cheese
- 8 celery stalks

Instructions:

1. Boil eggs for 9 minutes and let them cool
2. Peel and dice the eggs
3. Chop the cooked chicken finely
4. Slice celery into 2-inch-long pieces
5. Take a bowl and add all of the ingredients except celery
6. Mix well
7. Fill the celery sticks with the mixture and serve with more hot sauce
8. Enjoy!

Nutritional Information:

Calories per serving: 286, Fat: 20g, Carbohydrates: 2g, Protein: 19g

Choco Berry Protein Bars

(Total time: 15 mins.| Serves: 2)

Ingredients:

- ½ c. sliced almonds
- 1 c. chocolate protein powder
- ½ c. pecan pieces
- ½ c. fresh cherries
- ¼ c. fresh blueberries
- ¼ c. unsweetened coconut
- ½ c. almond butter
- ¼ c. coconut oil
- ¼ c. almond meal
- 1 tsp. vanilla
- 2 whole eggs
- ½ tsp. salt

Instructions:

1. Take a loaf pan and grease it
2. Pre-heat your oven to 325-degree Fahrenheit
3. Take a bowl and add all of the listed ingredients except fruit
4. Fold in berries and cherries into the batter
5. Pour into the pan
6. Bake for 10 minutes
7. Let it cool for 10 minutes
8. Cut into 12 bars and enjoy!

Nutritional Information:

Calories per serving: 235, Fat: 17, Carbohydrates: 6g, Protein: 8g

Amazing Chipotle Kale Chips

(Total time: 35 mins.| Serves: 4)

Ingredients:

- 2 large bunch kale
- 1 tbsp. olive oil
- 1/8 tsp. salt
- 1 tsp. chipotle powder
- ¼ c. parmesan cheese

Instructions:

1. Wash the kale thoroughly and dry them, cut into 4-inch pieces
2. Pre-heat your oven to 250-degree Fahrenheit
3. Take 3 baking sheets and line the with parchment paper
4. Take a bowl and add kale, coat with olive oil, cheese and chipotle
5. Place on baking sheet
6. Bake for 19 minutes and check crispiness
7. Bake for 9 minutes more if needed
8. Enjoy!

Nutritional Information:

Calories per serving: 37, Fat: 3g, Carbohydrates: 3g, Protein: 1g

Simple Fine Granola

(Total time: 16 mins.| Serves: 4)

Ingredients:

- 1 oz. cocao Sacha Inchi Seeds
- 1 oz. gureyere cheese, finely chopped
- 1 oz. pepitas, roasted

Instructions:

1. Take a zip bag and add all of the listed ingredients
2. Mix well and serve
3. Enjoy!

Nutritional Information:

Calories per serving: 449, Fat: 34g, Carbohydrates: 3g, Protein:25 g

Raspberry and Cheesy Pops

(Total time: 20 mins.| Serves: 8)

Ingredients:

- ¼ c. cream cheese
- ¼ c. chopped raspberries
- 4 tbsps. coconut oil
- 4 tbsps. heavy cream
- 4 tbsps. butter
- 1 tsp. vanilla extract

Instructions:

1. Add cream cheese, coconut oil, butter in a bowl

2. Mix well and microwave in 10 seconds interval until the cheese has melted

3. Remove the bowl and stir

4. Stir in heavy cream and fold in chopped raspberries

5. Stir in vanilla extra into the mix and stir

6. Pour the mix into ice cube tray for 16 sections Chill for 2 hours and serve!

Nutritional Information:

Calories per serving: 166, Fat: 17g, Carbohydrates: 2g, Protein: 0.8g

Buffalo Drumsticks

(Total time: 50 mins.| Serves: 4)

Ingredients:

- 2 lbs. chicken wings
- 2 tbsps. olive oil
- 2 tbsps. white wine vinegar
- 1 tbsp. tomato paste
- 1 tsp. salt
- 1 tsp. paprika powder
- 1 tbsp. tabasco

For Chili Aioli

- 2/3 c. mayonnaise
- 1 tbsp. smoked paprika
- 1 minced garlic clove

Instructions:

1. Pre-heat your oven to 450-degree Fahrenheit
2. Put drumstick in plastic bag
3. Mix the other ingredients in a bowl and pour the marinade into the plastic bag
4. Shake the bag well and allow the chicken to marinate for 10 minutes
5. Take a baking dish and coat it with oil
6. Transfer drumstick to baking dish and bake for 30-40 minutes
7. Take another bowl and mix aioli ingredients, serve with drumstick!
8. If you want, then you include some cucumber and carrot sticks as well!

Nutritional Information:

Calories per serving: 368, Fat: 18g, Carbohydrates: 8g, Protein: 42g

Satisfying Tuna Croquettes

(Total time: 15 mins.| Serves: 4)

Ingredients:

- 1 can of tuna, drained
- 1 whole large egg
- 8 tbsps. grated parmesan cheese
- 2 tbsps. flax meal
- Dash of salt
- Dash of pepper
- 1 tbsp. minced onion

Instructions:

1. Using a blender, mix all the ingredients (except flax meal) and pulse them mixture into a crunchy texture

2. Form patties using the mixture

3. Dip both sides of the patties in flax meals and fry them in hot oil until both sides are browned well

Nutritional Information:

Calories per serving: 105, Fat: 5g, Carbohydrates: 2g, Protein: 14g

Deep Walnut Bites

(Total time: 18 mins.| Serves: 10)

Ingredients:

- 6 oz. grated Parmesan cheese
- 2 tbsps. chopped walnuts
- 1 tbsp. unsalted butter
- ½ tbsp. chopped fresh thyme

Instructions:

1. Pre-heat your oven to 350-degree Fahrenheit
2. Take two large rimmed baking sheets and line with baking paper
3. Add parmesan cheese, butter to a food processor and blend
4. Add walnuts to the mixture and pulse
5. Take a tablespoon and scoop mix onto the baking sheet
6. Top with chopped thyme
7. Bake for 8 minutes and transfer to cooling rack
8. Let it cool for 30 minutes
9. Serve and enjoy!

Nutritional Information:

Calories per serving: 80, Fat: 3g, Carbohydrates: 7g, Protein: 7g

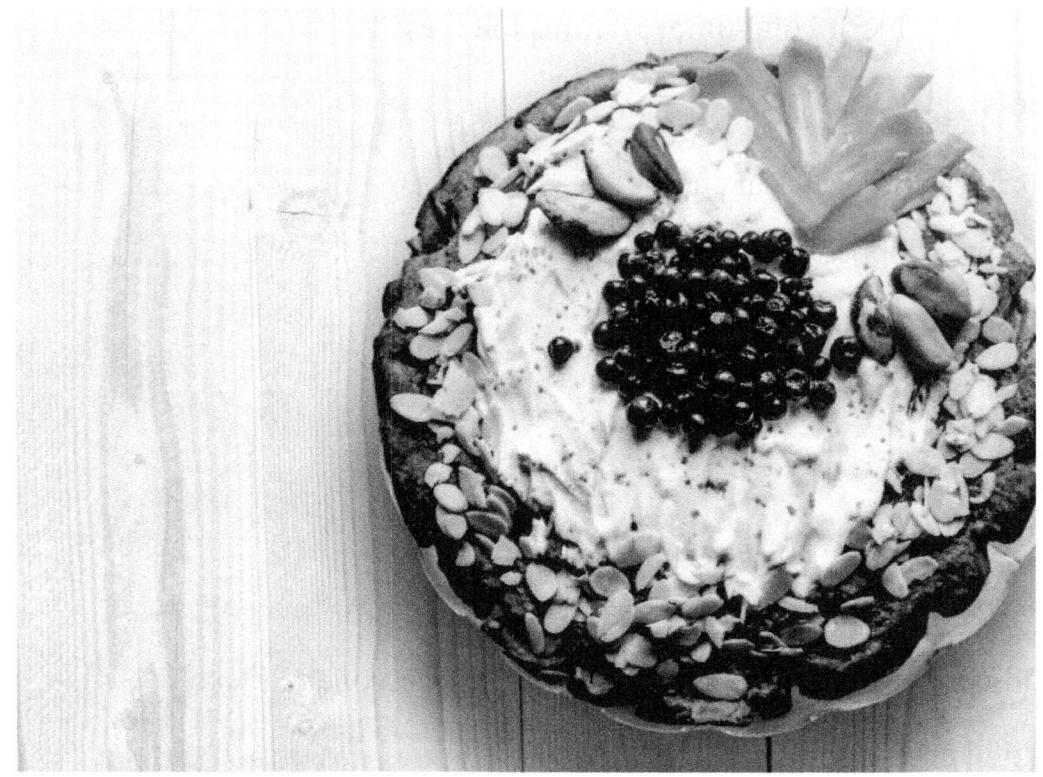

Pumpkin and Cardamom Donuts

(Total time: 32 mins.| Serves: 4)

Ingredients:

- 3 whole large eggs

- 1 c. pumpkin puree

- ½ c. coconut flour

- 1/3 c. melted butter

- 2 tbsps. erythritol

- 1 tsp. Cardamom

- ½ tsp. liquid stevia

- ¼ tsp. vanilla extract

- ¼ tsp. orange extract

- ¼ tsp. salt

Instructions:

1. Pre-heat your oven to 325-degree Fahrenheit

2. Take a microwave proof bowl and add butter and microwave the butter

3. Fold in the wet ingredients and mix

4. Take another bowl and add the dry ingredients, mix well and transfer the dry ingredients to the wet ingredients and mix

5. Roll up the dough into balls and place them in a cupcake tray

6. Bake for 20 minutes until slightly browned

7. Once cooled, dust with cinnamon and sweetener with a bit of maple syrup

8. Enjoy!

Nutritional Information:

Calories per serving: 149, Fat: 9g, Carbohydrates: 10g, Protein: 1g

Blueberry Morning Scones

(Total time: 25 mins.| Serves: 12)

Ingredients:

- 3 large eggs, beaten
- 1½ c. almond flour
- ¾ c. fresh/frozen raspberries
- ½ c. stevia
- 2 tsps. pure vanilla extract
- 2 tsps. baking powder

Instructions:

1. Pre-heat your oven to 375-degree Fahrenheit

2. Take a baking sheet and carefully line it with baking paper, keep the prepared sheet on the side

3. Take a large mixing bowl and add eggs, stevia, vanilla extract, baking powder and almond flour

4. Whisk the mixture well

5. Fold in raspberries and stir

6. Scoop the batter onto your baking sheet and make mounds (keep 2 inch distance between each mound)

7. Bake for 15 minutes and transfer to cooling rack

8. Let them cool for 10 minutes

9. Enjoy!

Nutritional Information:

Calories per serving: 133, Fat: 8g, Carbohydrates: 4g, Protein: 2g

Deliciously Chocolate Coated Bacon

(Total time: 35 mins.| Serves: 6)

Ingredients:

- 12 bacon slices
- 4½ tbsps. unsweetened dark chocolate
- 2¼ tbsps. coconut oil
- 1½ tsp. liquid stevia

Instructions:

1. Pre-heat your oven to 425-degree Fahrenheit
2. Skewer bacon into iron skewers
3. Arrange the skewers on a baking sheet
4. Bake for 15 minutes until crispy
5. Transfer to cooling rack
6. Take a saucepan and place it over low heat, add coconut oil and melt it
7. Stir in chocolate and melt
8. Add stevia and stir
9. Place crispy bacon on a sheet of parchment paper and coat with chocolate mix
10. Let the chocolate dry and serve
11. Enjoy!

Nutritional Information:

Calories per serving: 258, Fat: 26g, Carbohydrates: 0.5g, Protein: 7g

Easy Bake Coconut Macaroons

(Total time: 2hrs 20 mins.| Serves: 18)

Ingredients:

- 1½ c. shredded unsweetened coconut

- ¾ c. unsweetened coconut milk

- 2¼ tsps. stevia

Instructions:

1. Add the listed ingredients to a bowl

2. Mix them well and tightly cover the mixture with plastic wrap

3. Refrigerate for 2 hours

4. Once chilled, scoop the coconut mix into balls and serve!

Nutritional Information:

Calories per serving: 47, Fat: 5g, Carbohydrates: 2g, Protein: 0.4g

Poppy Seed Juicy Cupcake

(Total time: 35 mins.| Serves: 4)

Ingredients:

- ¾ c. Blanched Almond flour
- ¼ c. Golden Flaxseed Meal
- 1/3 c. Erythritol
- 1 tsp. baking powder
- 2 tbsps. Poppy Seeds
- ¼ c. salted butter
- ¼ c. heavy cream
- 3 large eggs
- 2 lemons
- 3 tbsps. lemon juice
- 1 tsp. vanilla extract
- 25 drops of liquid stevia

Instructions:

1. Pre-heat your oven to 350-degree Fahrenheit
2. Take a mixing bowl and add poppy seeds, almond flour and Erythritol
3. Add Flaxseed meal and stir
4. Add melted butter and pour heavy cream
5. Add egg and mix well
6. Pour batter into cupcake molds and bake for 20 minutes
7. Cool for 10 minutes and enjoy!

Nutritional Information:

Calories per serving: 229, Fat: 15g, Carbohydrates: 14g, Protein: 6g

Raspberry Popsicles

(Total time: 2 hrs.| Serves: 4)

Ingredients:

- 3½ oz. Raspberries
- ½ lemon
- ¼ c. coconut oil
- 1 c. coconut milk
- ¼ c. sour cream
- ¼ c. heavy cream
- ½ tsp. Guar Gum
- 20 drops of Liquid Stevia

Instructions:

1. Take an immersion blender and toss in all of the ingredients and blend them altogether nicely

2. Once done, take them mixture through a mesh and strain the mixture, discarding all of the raspberry seeds

3. Pour in the mixture into a mold and keep the mold inside the fridge for 2 hours

4. Once done, pass the mold through hot water to dislodge the popsicles

Nutritional Information:

Calories per serving: 65, Fat: 1g, Carbohydrates: 8g, Protein: 3g

Secret Yogurt Parfait

(Total time: 10 mins.| Serves: 4)

Ingredients:

- 1 c. walnuts
- Sweetener
- 1 c. shredded coconut
- 2 c. full fat yogurt
- 4 handful blueberries
- 4 handful strawberries
- 4 bananas
- 1 c. toasted flax seeds
- 1 c. Macadamia pieces

Instructions:

1. Take a mason jar and add 3 tablespoons of yogurt to the bottom

2. Add sweetener then make layers of nuts, coconut and bananas, making sure to keep alternating between ingredients while making the layers

3. Pour the remaining yogurt on top

4. Enjoy!

Nutritional Information:

Calories per serving: 230, Fat: 15g, Carbohydrates: 9g, Protein: 20g

Choco Peanut Fat Bombs

(Total time: 1 hr. 15 mins.| Serves: 8)

Ingredients:

- 2 tbsps. butter

- 2 tbsps. coconut oil

- 2 tbsps. heavy cream

- 1 tbsp. smooth peanut butter

- 1 tbsp. unsweetened cocoa powder

- ½ tsp. vanilla extract

- ½ tsp. liquid stevia

Instructions:

1. Add peanut butter, coconut oil, butter in a microwave proof bowl and microwave in 10 second intervals until fully melted

2. Stir the mix and add heavy cream and mix

3. Add cocoa powder, vanilla extract and stevia and stir

4. Pour the mix into ice cube tray with 8 chambers and freeze for 1 hour

5. Serve and enjoy!

Nutritional Information:

Calories per serving: 73, Fat: 8g, Carbohydrates: 1g, Protein: 0.6g

Creamy Vanilla Pudding

(Total time: 17 mins.| Serves: 4)

Ingredients:

- 2 large egg yolks

- 1 c. heavy cream

- 1½ tsp. stevia

- 1 tsp. arrowroot flour

- ½ tsp. pure vanilla extract

- Sea salt

Instructions:

1. Take a heavy-duty saucepan and add egg yolks

2. Whisk in cream, stevia, arrowroot flour, pure vanilla extract and mix well

3. Season with salt and whisk

4. Place it over medium heat and stir until the mixture just starts to steam

5. Lower heat to low and keep stirring for 10 minutes

6. Pour pudding into 4 heatproof containers

7. Serve and enjoy!

Nutritional Information:

Calories per serving: 135, Fat: 13g, Carbohydrates: 2g, Protein: 2g

Pretty Pizza Fat Bombs

(Total time: 10 mins.| Serves: 6)

Ingredients:

- 4 oz. Cream cheese

- 14 slices of peperoni

- 8 pitted of black olives

- 2 tbsps. Sun dried tomato pesto

- 2 tbsps. Chopped basil

- Salt

- Pepper

Instructions:

1. Dice up your olives and pepperonis into small sized portions

2. Add the rest of the ingredients in a bowl alongside the cut-up pieces and toss everything well

3. Form balls using the mixture and garnish with some olive, basil and pepperoni

4. Serve!

Nutritional Information:

Calories per serving: 28, Fat: 3g, Carbohydrates: 0g, Protein: 1g

14-Days Keto Meal Plan for Rapid Fat Loss With 2-Weeks Healthy Shopping List

Day 1

Breakfast: Sausage and Egg Muffin

Lunch: Buffalo Chicken Lettuce Wraps

Dinner: Cauliflower taboule salad

Snack: Herb Dressed Chicken Parmesan Fingers

Dessert: Pumpkin and Cardamom Donuts

Day 2

Breakfast: Breakfast Loaf with Berry and Peanut Butter

Lunch: Vegetarian Cauliflower Curry

Dinner: Thai Chicken with cauliflower rice

Snack: Bacon Moza Sticks

Dessert: Blueberry Morning Scones

Day 3

Breakfast: Keto Cereal

Lunch: Beef Burritos

Dinner: Spinach salad with bacon and blue cheese

Snack: Buffalo Chicken Dip

Dessert: Deliciously Chocolate Coated Bacon

Day 4

Breakfast: Ham and Cheese Waffles

Lunch: Open-Faced Prosciutto and Brie Sandwich with Avocado Bun

Dinner: Grilled chicken skewers with garlic sauce

Snack: Choco Berry Protein Bars

Dessert: Easy Bake Coconut Macaroons

Day 5

Breakfast: Baked Eggs with Avocado

Lunch: Keto Cubano

Dinner: Pasta with chicken and basil

Snack: Amazing Chipotle Kale Chips

Dessert: Poppy Seed Juicy Cupcake

Day 6

Breakfast: Sausage and Egg Muffin

Lunch: Open-Faced Prosciutto and Brie Sandwich with Avocado Bun

Dinner: Cauliflower taboule salad

Snack: Bacon Moza Sticks

Dessert: Pumpkin and Cardamom Donuts

Day 7

Breakfast: Ham and Cheese Waffles

Lunch: Vegetarian Cauliflower Curry

Dinner: Spinach salad with bacon and blue cheese

Snack: Choco Berry Protein Bars

Dessert: Poppy Seed Juicy Cupcake

Day 8

Breakfast: Cheese, Egg and Bacon Cups

Lunch: Keto Monkey Bread

Dinner: Salmon Fishcakes

Snack: Simple Fine Granola

Dessert: Raspberry Popsicles

Day 9

Breakfast: Yoghurt Parfait

Lunch: Cauliflower Grits With Roasted Mushrooms And Walnuts

Dinner: Baby back Ribs

Snack: Raspberry and Cheesy Pops

Dessert: Secret Yogurt Parfait

Day 10

Breakfast: Salad with chicken breast and spinach

Lunch: Spicy Roast Beef Cups

Dinner: Garlic Cream Pork Chops

Snack: Buffalo Drumsticks

Dessert: Choco Peanut Fat Bombs

Day 11

Breakfast: Bacon lemon thyme breakfast muffins

Lunch: Crispy Pork Salad

Dinner: Spaghetti Carbonara

Snack: Satisfying Tuna Croquettes

Dessert: Creamy Vanilla Pudding

Day 12

Breakfast: Cheese omelet with bacon

Lunch: Goat Cheese and Vegetable Salad

Dinner: Shrimp in Tuscan Cream Sauce

Snack: Deep Walnut Bites

Dessert: Pretty Pizza Fat Bombs

Day 13

Breakfast: Salad with chicken breast and spinach

Lunch: Spicy Roast Beef Cups

Dinner: Salmon Fishcakes

Snack: Buffalo Drumsticks

Dessert: Secret Yogurt Parfait

Day 14

Breakfast: Cheese omelet with bacon

Lunch: Crispy Pork Salad

Dinner: Garlic Cream Pork Chops

Snack: Satisfying Tuna Croquettes

Dessert: Creamy Vanilla Pudding

Week One Meal plan and shopping list

- Eggs
- butter
- Avocado
- berries
- spices
- seasonings
- milk
- coconut
- flax seeds
- nuts
- cheese
- chicken
- lime
- tomatoes
- sesame seeds
- ham
- pork
- lemon
- sunflower oil
- almonds
- kale

Week two Meal Plan and shopping list

- eggs
- bacon
- spinach
- seasonings - salt, pepper
- nuts
- yoghurt
- bananas
- berries
- macadamia
- chicken
- olive oil
- lemon

- ghee
- beef
- mushrooms
- salmon
- coconut

- shirataki noodles
- shrimp
- tomatoes
- kale
- flax seeds

Conclusion

Once again, I would like to thank you for choosing this book and having the patience of reading it. I do hope you had as much fun reading and experimenting with the recipes as much I enjoyed preparing the book for you. You can use a ketogenic diet just to improve health and not necessarily to lose weight, of course.

Keto is a lifesaver for many people. It is nice to feel satisfied, to eat delicious food and still to lose weight. Keep in mind: the more physical training and activity you have, the faster fat burns.

-- [Kathy Robinson]

Made in the USA
Middletown, DE
29 November 2018